BEAT ANXIETY AND DEPRESSION WITH DIET.

Karen Reynolds

USUALLY NOT THE ONLY HEALTH ISSUE.

About ten years ago I started to suffer with anxiety and depression. It was not my only health problem and I soon realised that I had a growing list of other health problems that came along with it. If you suffer from anxiety and/or depression it will probably not be your only symptom either. You will also be more likely to suffer from other health problems such as these:

Food allergies or intolerances.

Hay fever.

Irritable bowel syndrome.

Rashes.

Sensitive skin.

Constipation.

Bloating.

Indigestion.

Headaches.

Migraines.

Fatigue.

Hyperactivity and nervousness.

Forgetfulness.

Depression.

Acne.

Eczema.

Asthma.

Psoriasis.

Difficultly sleeping.

Difficulty concentrating.

Muscle spasms and tics.

Muscle cramps and stiffness.

Weak nails that break easily.

Hair that is brittle with split ends.

Heart burn.

Loss of appetite.

Feeling nauseous.

Frequent colds and viruses.

Restless leg syndrome.

High blood pressure.

High cholesterol.

Sweating more than usual with a stronger odour.

Seizures.

Dizziness.

Loss of balance.

Palpitations.

Panic attacks.

Over thinking.

Karen Reynolds

Brain fog.

Clumsiness.

Lack of coordination.

Irritable bowel syndrome.

MY PLAN OF ACTION.

I did the normal things that most people do – went to the doctor etc but none of the medications they suggested really helped at all and they all made me feel worse. I looked online and found a good Naturopath out of desperation and similarly had no improvement with their suggested treatments either. I spent loads of money on the high strength friendly bacteria and probiotic capsules they advised me to take but nothing made any difference, in fact the probiotics made me feel quite ill. Interestingly I noticed that the more powerful - higher the strength, the probiotics were the worse I felt after taking them.

I also tried homeopathy and acupuncture and ended up spending a lot of money on that too with no improvement. I tried doing the candida diet which didn't help either. Basically I was willing to try almost anything to see if it could help.

The last treatment I tried was vitamin and mineral therapy. This involved sending off a sample of my hair which the company would analyse. They then sent me a list of vitamins and minerals that they recommended me to take. I again spent a lot of money buying all the vitamins and minerals that had been recommended and was taking about six tablets twice a day of high strength vitamin C, calcium and vit D, vitamin B complex and vitamin E. After a few days I had to stop that treatment due to bad stomach pains and diarreah.

I soon realised that I was going to have to help myself and started to do some research online. I discovered that there were lots of other people out there also suffering with similar problems. One day I googled a list of all my symptoms and 'lack of magnesium' appeared as one of the suggested causes. I started to read books on magnesium and look at websites about magnesium. When I started to look at the functions of magnesium in the body it all started to make sense. Magnesium is responsible for about three hundred biochemical reactions in the human body. I will list the main ones in the next chapter.

ROLES OF MAGNESIUM IN THE HUMAN BODY.

Energy production – magnesium is needed to metabolise proteins, fats and carbohydrates - helps to beat fatigue.

Mood regulation – helps depression and mood swings.

Brain function – concentration, memory.

Muscle movements – helps muscle cramps and stiffness.

Nervous system regulation – helps reduce anxiety – keeps you calm.

Immune system function – helps to keep your immune system working properly.

Bone health – you need magnesium to help you absorb calcium, they work together in tandem.

Production of enzymes – helps manufacture digestive enzymes so therefore helps with digestion.

Helps adjust blood glucose levels – keeps blood sugar levels stable and prevents diabetes.

Detoxification of cells – helps to detox the body and takes toxic metals caused by pollution out of the body: Lead, cadmium, aluminium.

Helps regulate blood pressure.

Helps with heart health - needed for proper heart rhythm.

Helps regulate cholesterol levels.

Cell regulation and reproduction.

Cancer prevention – in a study that was done in Paris men that had the highest magnesium consumption slashed their risk of getting cancer by fifty per cent.

Reduces gall stone formation.

Protects our DNA.

RESEARCHING HIGH MAGNESIUM FOODS.

Then I found some websites that contained good nutritional information and started to look at which foods were the highest in magnesium. I made a list and started to include the foods I liked from it in my diet. I didn't expect any immediate improvements but even on the first day I noticed a difference.I noticed an improvement in how I felt physically and mentally. My symptoms improved dramatically so I continued with the high magnesium diet and have done so ever since.

Improvements I noticed and to look for are :

Better sleep.

More energy.

Better mood and feeling of wellbeing.

Less depressed.

Calmer and less anxious.

Having more regular bowel movements.

Better skin and less acne.

Better concentration.

Better memory.

Feeling less distracted.

Improvement in bloating.

Flatter stomach.

Less indigestion.

Improvement in PMS symptoms.

Increase in appetite.

Feeling more alert.

Feeling less stressed and panicky.

Less headaches.

PMS symptoms improved.

Big improvement in Irritable bowel syndrome.

Better coordination.

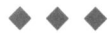

HIGH MAGNESIUM FOODS TO INCLUDE IN YOUR DIET

Avoid all foods you are allergic too, are intolerant to or do not like! Only pick foods from the list you enjoy eating so you will stick to it long-term.

Cocoa powder or anything containing it:

Chocolate (not white chocolate), chocolate cake, chocolate wholegrain biscuits, flapjack.

Chocolate covered nuts

Chocolate covered raisins

Chocolate spread

Chocolate wholegrain cereal

Seaweed

Herbs – dried or fresh – coriander, dill, chives, parsley, mint, basil, sage, tarragon.

Spices – turmeric, cumin, black pepper, cardamom, curry powder.

Nuts, nut butter: peanuts, almonds, cashews, hazelnuts.

Seeds – pumpkin seeds, sunflower seeds, sesame seeds.

Green vegetables – spinach, broccoli, sugar snaps, asparagus, avocado, lettuce, kale, dark green cabbage, green beans, cucumber with skin.

Wholemeal/wholegrain bread, rye bread.

Whole wheat pitta bread.

Whole wheat wraps.

Wholegrain bread sticks.

Wholemeal crackers, corn crackers, oatcakes, rice crackers, buckwheat crackers.

Popcorn.

Sweet corn

Mushrooms

Olives

Whole wheat pasta

Buckwheat pasta

Spelt pasta

Wholegrains – oats, corn, spelt, rye, barley, brown rice, buckwheat.

Pulses – chickpeas, lentils, quinoa, all beans, peas, split peas.

Hummus, guacamole.

Fruit – Apples with skin, bananas, watermelon, passion fruit.

Drinks - Tea, coffee, hot chocolate, chocolate milkshake, green tea, mint tea, nettle tea, water.

Sweet snacks – flapjacks, chocolate, chocolate cake/brownies, wholegrain cereal bars, wholegrain chocolate biscuits/ cookies: Hobnobs, Digestives.

Potatoes with their skin on: Jacket potato or potato wedges (the majority of the magnesium in a potato is in the skin.)

Sweet potato wedges with skins on.

Fish – tuna, salmon, mackerel, prawns, crab, lobster, herring, halibut

Lentil crisps.

Chickpea crisps.

FOODS AND THINGS TO AVOID ON THE DIET

*All the following things help to
deplete your magnesium.*

White flour in any form – white bread, crackers that are not wholegrain (all the magnesium in grains are in their outershell.)

Refined white sugar and salt.

Sugary coloured sweets.

Crisps – these are loaded with salt and fat and are made with potatoes without their skins on.

Sugary drinks – pop, squash, cordials, fruit juice.

Chips, fries and mashed potato - very low in magnesium as practically all the magnesium is in the skin of the potato.

Cut down on alcohol, smoking, drugs.

Stress also depletes your magnesium levels – so try to eliminate any unnecessary sources of stress in your life.

Relax – make time to relax each day and do something you enjoy. A walk in the countryside, a walk with the dog. Painting, reading, singing or gardening. Anything you find therapeutic will help you destress.

Wear gloves when using chemical cleaners so it doesn't absorb into your skin and therefore into your bloodstream.

Not getting enough sleep.

Radiation - too much time spent in front of computer screens. Too much sun exposure.

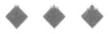

START BY MAKING SMALL CHANGES

Choose items from the list that you like and enjoy eating. Try to include at least one item containing magnesium at each meal and snack and then start to gradually experiment and increase until you have a few items at each meal containing magnesium.

Look at the list of high magnesium foods for inspiration on new food combinations and meals. If you have time and are good at cooking you could even make your own wholemeal pastry and make some high magnesium pies and pasties for a change. There is always a way of making a high magnesium version of most things.

Don't be put off by whole wheat pasta. You can hardly tell the difference. I particularly like the wholemeal spaghetti and fusilli. Herbs are very high in magnesium so adding a few dried herbs to a meal will significantly increase the magnesium content.

Dairy products are much higher in calcium than magnesium so adding cocoa powder to them will really boost their magnesium content and help you to absorb all the calcium properly. Hot chocolate and chocolate milkshake are ideal drinks because of this.

Likewise cheese and chives are a good combination as the very high magnesium content of chives helps to balance out the very high calcium content of the cheese and so helps you to absorb all the calcium properly.

MEAL SUGGESTIONS

Breakfast ideas

Chocolate spread on wholemeal toast.

Chocolate wholegrain cereals with milk.

Whole grain cereal bar.

Chocolate porridge.

Sliced banana topped with yogurt and grated chocolate.

Porridge with maple syrup.

Avocado on wholegrain toast.

Hot chocolate and wholegrain toast with butter.

Wholegrain toast with nut butter (if not allergic to nuts).

Banana, nut and chocolate smoothie.

Banana, avocado and chocolate smoothie.

Whole wheat or buckwheat pancakes filled with sliced banana and chocolate spread.

Bacon, egg, beans, mushrooms with potato wedges (healthier alternative to a fried breakfast).

Mushroom omelette with chopped chives.

Wholemeal eggy bread.

Banana nut and chocolate muffin.

Chocolate protein shake.

Chocolate protein bar.

Granola.

Chocolate granola.

Muesli.

Chocolate chip and nut muesli.

Yogurt layered with sliced banana, muesli/granola and chocolate chips in a tall dessert dish.

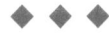

Snacks ideas

Chocolate bar.

Chocolate nut bar.

Cereal bar.

Banana.

Apple with skin on.

Wholegrain chocolate biscuits.

Whole wheat or oat biscuits or cookies.

Chocolate cake or brownie.

Flapjack or chocolate covered flapjack.

Corn chips.

Lentil crisps.

Chickpea crisps.

Oatcakes or wholegrain crackers with chocolate spread.

Chocolate coated corn cakes.

Olives.

Wholemeal bread sticks with hummus.

Chocolate protein bar.

Nuts – peanuts, almonds, cashews, hazelnuts and pecans.

Chocolate covered nuts.

Chocolate covered raisins.

Granola.

Chocolate protein bar.

Lunch ideas

Wholemeal toasted pitta bread or wholemeal wrap filled with curry.

Hummus on oatcakes with salad.

Jacket potato with chilli con carne.

Jacket potato with tuna mayonnaise and sweet corn.

Wholegrain sandwich with salmon and cucumber.

Wholegrain sandwich with tuna mayo and sweetcorn.

Loaded potato wedges.

Mackerel pate on wholegrain toast or crackers.

Guacamole with corn chips.

Mushroom omelette.

Prawn and potato salad with chives and mayonnaise. Leave the skins on the potatoes.

Whole wheat base pizza with ham, cheese, mushroom and herb topping.

Whole wheat pitta bread with chicken and salad – include some green: lettuce, spinach, chives or cucumber.

Rye crackers or bread with sliced banana and chocolate spread.

Evening meal ideas

Risotto made with wholegrain rice.

Kedgeree – rice, turmeric, eggs and flaked mackerel.

Chilli with brown rice.

Salmon steak with potato wedges with broccoli.

Bolognaise with wholegrain pasta.

Tuna pasta bake with wholegrain pasta.

Salmon steak, asparagus spears and new potatoes with skins on.

Chicken and mushroom filled omelette with salad.

Chicken Kiev with potato wedges and peas.

Bean stew with brown rice or corn chips.

Ratatouille in a jacket potato.

Salmon and avocado salad.

Tuna and egg salad.

Curry (vegetarian, meat or fish) with wholemeal pitta bread and brown rice.

Pakoras – gram four (chickpea flour) mixed with turmeric and other herbs and spices, sliced vegetables then fried).

Onion bhajis – also made with gram flour and turmeric, so high in magnesium.

Desserts

Chocolate cheesecake.

Chocolate ice cream with chocolate chips.

Banoffee pie sprinkled with grated chocolate.

Chocolate ice-cream sprinkled with nuts and sliced banana.

Chocolate brownies.

Chocolate fudge cake.

Apple or any other fruit crumble made with whole wheat and oat topping.

Banana surprise - Sliced bananas drizzled with melted chocolate, chopped nuts, whipped cream and topped with grated chocolate – layer it up into a tall glass dessert dish (add ice cream if desired.)

Avocado chocolate mousse – blend avocado, cocoa powder, maple syrup and bananas together and chill in fridge.

Chocolate custard – just add some cocoa powder to normal custard.

Chocolate crispy cakes – mix melted chocolate with cornflakes, form into clumps and leave to set in the fridge. Add raisins or chopped or flaked nuts to the mix to customise to your taste.

Wholemeal pancakes filled with sliced banana and drizzled with melted chocolate. Mix cream with melted chocolate to make a quick chocolate sauce.

Chocolate tiffin squares.

Rocky road.

Chocolate muffins.

If you have a waffle maker you could make a wholemeal batter and make wholemeal waffles for dessert or breakfast.

TAKING A MAGNESIUM SUPPLEMENT INSTEAD.

The more health problems you have off the list at the beginning of this book, the more deficient in magnesium you will be. If you find you cannot get enough improvement with the diet alone you could try taking a magnesium supplement as well.

Or if you just don't like a lot of the foods on the diet or are intolerant or allergic to them, then just taking a good quality magnesium supplement could be an option for you. I also do this sometimes if I have been out and eaten junk food or been to a party and have eaten badly. I have found magnesium citrate to be the best form to take as it is easily absorbed. I started off with a low dose and gradually increased until I achieved a perfect bowel movement every day. Keep a note of how much you are taking in a diary or on your calendar. Too much magnesium will make your bowel movements too loose and too little magnesium will leave you constipated.

Everyone is different and therefore will need a different amount of magnesium daily. Finding your own personal dose that works for you is the most important thing. Just experiment until you get it right.

Your personal dose will be the dose that makes you do a normal bowel movement daily. Spreading the dose into smaller doses over the day and taking a bit every time you eat will make you feel much better than taking the whole dose in one go.

This is because magnesium is needed to digest proteins, fats and carbohydrates so is therefore needed and most important at mealtimes to help you digest your food properly and therefore give you energy from it.

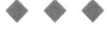